Methylene Blue

Methylene Blue as a Neuroprotective Agent

By

Glasser Blake

Table of Contents

CHAPTER 1

How was Methylene Blue Found

Methylene blue is a synthetic dye that has been used for various purposes since its discovery in the late 19th century. The compound has a complex history, with many different scientists and industries contributing to its development and use over the years. To understand how methylene blue was found, we need to delve into the history of synthetic dyes and the chemical industry of the 19th century.

The development of synthetic dyes can be traced back to the mid-19th century, when chemists began experimenting with coal tar as a potential source of new chemical compounds. Coal tar is a byproduct of the coal gasification process, and it contains a complex mixture of organic compounds that were largely unexplored at the time. In 1856, a young British chemist named William Perkin accidentally discovered the first synthetic dye while attempting to synthesize quinine, a medication for malaria. Perkin's experiment produced a purple substance that he later identified as aniline purple, which was later renamed mauveine.

Perkin's discovery sparked a flurry of activity in the synthetic dye industry, as chemists around the world began experimenting with coal tar and other organic sources to create new dyes. By the 1870s, the industry had grown into a major economic force, with companies like BASF and Bayer leading the way in the development of new dyes and pigments.

One of the scientists who played a significant role in the development of synthetic dyes was Heinrich Caro, a German chemist who worked for BASF.

Caro was a talented chemist who had already made important contributions to the chemical industry, including the discovery of a new process for producing sulfuric acid. In the late 1870s, Caro began working on a new synthetic dye that would become known as methylene blue.

The exact circumstances of Caro's discovery are unclear, but it is believed that he was inspired by the work of other chemists who had synthesized related compounds. Methylene blue is a member of the phenothiazine family of compounds, which includes several other dyes and medications with similar structures. One of the most notable members of this family is chlorpromazine, which was later developed as an antipsychotic medication.

Caro's work on methylene blue was initially focused on its use as a dye for textiles and other materials. The compound was found to produce a vivid blue color that was resistant to fading and had good staining properties. However, it was soon discovered that methylene blue had other properties that made it useful for a variety of other applications.

One of the earliest medical uses of methylene blue was as a treatment for malaria. In the early 1890s, a German physician named Paul Ehrlich began experimenting with methylene blue as a way to kill the parasites that caused the disease. Ehrlich found that methylene blue was effective at killing the parasites in laboratory experiments, and he went on to conduct clinical trials with human patients. Although methylene blue was not as effective as quinine, which was the standard treatment for malaria at the time, it was still useful in certain cases and helped pave the way for other antimalarial drugs.

Methylene blue also had other medical uses, including as a treatment for cyanide poisoning and as a diagnostic tool for certain conditions. In the early 20th century, methylene blue was used as a stain in microscopy to help identify certain types of bacteria and other microorganisms. It was also used in a variety of other industrial and scientific applications, including as a dye for histological specimens, as a marker in DNA sequencing, and as a tool for studying mitochondrial function.

In the decades since its discovery, methylene blue has continued to be used for a wide range of purposes. It has been the subject of extensive research in the fields of medicine, biology, chemistry, and materials science, and new applications for the compound are still being discovered today. For example, recent studies have shown that methylene blue may be useful in the treatment of Alzheimer's disease and other neurodegenerative disorders, as well as in the treatment of certain types of cancer.

The discovery of methylene blue is a testament to the ingenuity and creativity of scientists working in the chemical industry of the 19th century. Although the compound was initially developed as a textile dye, its unique properties and versatility made it a valuable tool in a variety of other fields. Today, methylene blue remains an important compound in both industry and scientific research, and its legacy serves as a reminder of the power of innovation and discovery in driving progress and advancing knowledge.

CHAPTER 2

Harmful Effect of Methylene Blue

Methylene blue is generally considered safe when used as directed, but like any medication or chemical compound, it can have harmful effects if used improperly or in excessive amounts. In this answer, we will explore the potential harmful effects of methylene blue, including its toxicity, side effects, and interactions with other medications.

Toxicity: Methylene blue is considered to have low toxicity when used as directed, but in large amounts, it can be toxic. The LD50 (the dose at which 50% of test animals die) for methylene blue in rats is around 1000mg/kg of body weight, which means that a lethal dose for a human could be as little as 70-150mg/kg. However, it's important to note that these values can vary depending on factors such as age, health status, and individual sensitivity.

Acute toxicity from methylene blue ingestion is rare, but it can occur if large amounts are consumed. Symptoms of acute toxicity may include nausea, vomiting, abdominal pain, dizziness, confusion, and methemoglobinemia (a condition in which red blood cells are unable to transport oxygen effectively). In severe cases, methylene blue toxicity can lead to seizures, coma, and death.

Side Effects: When used as directed, methylene blue is generally well-tolerated, but some people may experience side effects. Common side effects of methylene blue include:

- Blue or green discoloration of urine, stool, or skin (temporary)

- Headache

- Dizziness

- Nausea or vomiting

- Abdominal pain or discomfort

- Shortness of breath

- Blurred vision or changes in color perception

- Fatigue or weakness

These side effects are generally mild and go away on their own after treatment is discontinued. However, if you experience any of these symptoms while taking methylene blue, it's important to consult your healthcare provider to rule out any underlying health conditions.

Interactions: Methylene blue can interact with certain medications, which can increase the risk of harmful side effects. Some of the medications that may interact with methylene blue include:

- Serotonin reuptake inhibitors (SSRIs): Methylene blue can increase the risk of serotonin syndrome when taken with SSRIs, which can cause symptoms such as agitation, confusion, rapid heartbeat, high blood pressure, and seizures.

- Monoamine oxidase inhibitors (MAOIs): Methylene blue can

increase the risk of hypertensive crisis when taken with MAOIs, which can cause a sudden increase in blood pressure and potentially life-threatening complications.

- Benzodiazepines: Methylene blue can decrease the effectiveness of benzodiazepines, which are commonly used to treat anxiety and insomnia.

- Opioids: Methylene blue can increase the risk of respiratory depression when taken with opioids, which can cause breathing difficulties and potentially

life-threatening
complications.

Methylene blue may also interact with other medications or supplements, so it's important to consult with your healthcare provider before taking methylene blue if you're currently taking any other medications or supplements.

There are other possible adverse reactions to methylene blue, including allergic reactions and interactions with certain medical conditions.

Allergic reactions: Although rare, some people may develop an allergic reaction to methylene blue. Symptoms of an allergic reaction may include skin rash, itching, swelling of the face or tongue, difficulty breathing, or chest pain. If you experience any of these symptoms, seek medical attention immediately.

Medical conditions: Methylene blue should be used with caution or avoided in people with certain medical conditions. These include:

- G6PD deficiency: People with glucose-6-phosphate dehydrogenase (G6PD) deficiency should not take methylene blue, as it can cause a breakdown of red blood cells and lead to anemia.

- Renal impairment: Methylene blue is primarily excreted through the kidneys, so it should be used with caution or avoided in people with impaired kidney function.

- Hepatic impairment: Methylene blue is metabolized in the liver, so it should be used with caution or avoided in people with liver disease or impaired liver function.

- Cardiovascular disease: Methylene blue can increase blood pressure and heart rate, so it should be used with caution in people with cardiovascular disease or hypertension.

It's important to note that these are not all the potential harmful effects of methylene blue, and there may be other factors to consider based on individual circumstances. As with any medication or chemical compound, it's essential to use methylene blue only as directed by a healthcare provider, and to report any unusual symptoms or side effects immediately.

CHAPTER 3

Application and Uses of Methylene Blue

Methylene blue has a wide range of applications and uses across different fields, including medicine, biology, chemistry, and industrial processes. Its versatility is due to its unique chemical properties and ability to interact with a variety of molecules and structures.

In medicine, methylene blue has been used for over a century as a diagnostic and therapeutic agent. Here are some of the key

applications and uses of
methylene blue in medicine:

Diagnostic uses:

- Staining tissues: Methylene
  blue is commonly used to
  stain tissues in histology
  and pathology to aid in
  diagnosis and research.

- Visualization of anatomy:
  Methylene blue can be used
  to visualize the anatomy of
  certain structures in the
  body, such as the lymphatic
  system.

- Detection of leaks:
  Methylene blue can be used
  to detect leaks in certain
  surgical procedures, such as

the identification of a urinary leak after bladder surgery.

Therapeutic uses:

- Antimicrobial agent: Methylene blue has been shown to have antimicrobial properties, particularly against Gram-positive bacteria, and is used in the treatment of infections such as methicillin-resistant Staphylococcus aureus (MRSA).

- Treatment of methemoglobinemia: Methylene blue is a first-line treatment for methemoglobinemia, a condition in which the oxygen-carrying capacity of the blood is reduced due to the presence of methemoglobin.

- Treatment of malaria: Methylene blue has been used as an antimalarial drug, both alone and in combination with other medications.

- Treatment of vasoplegic syndrome: Methylene blue can be used to treat vasoplegic syndrome, a condition in which blood vessels become dilated and blood pressure drops during surgery or other medical procedures.

methylene blue also has applications in other fields, including:

Biology:

- Staining of cells and tissues: Methylene blue is used to stain cells and tissues in microscopy to visualize cellular structures and functions.

- Tracking of molecules: Methylene blue can be used as a tracer to track the movement of molecules within cells and tissues.

- Vital staining: Methylene blue can be used in vital staining, a technique in which living cells are stained to allow for visualization and analysis.

Chemistry:

- Redox indicator: Methylene blue can be used as a redox indicator in chemical reactions, as it changes color depending on the oxidation state of the reaction.

- Electrophoresis: Methylene blue can be used as a dye in gel electrophoresis to visualize DNA and protein molecules.

- Photodynamic therapy: Methylene blue can be used in photodynamic therapy, a cancer treatment that uses a combination of light and a photosensitizing agent to destroy cancer cells.

Industrial processes:

- Dyeing: Methylene blue is used as a dye in textiles and other materials.

- Water treatment: Methylene blue can be used in water treatment to remove certain pollutants and contaminants.

- Indicator: Methylene blue can be used as an indicator

in various industrial processes, such as in the production of sulfuric acid.

methylene blue is a versatile and widely used compound with a range of applications and uses in medicine, biology, chemistry, and industrial processes. Its properties and mechanisms of action make it useful for a variety of diagnostic, therapeutic, and research purposes, as well as in industrial applications.

While the uses of methylene blue outlined above are some of the most well-known and widely used, there are many other potential applications of this compound that are currently

being studied and developed.
Here are some examples:

Neuroprotective agent:
Methylene blue has been studied
for its potential as a
neuroprotective agent,
particularly in the treatment of
neurodegenerative diseases such
as Alzheimer's and Parkinson's.
Some research has suggested that
methylene blue may help to
prevent the accumulation of
amyloid-beta plaques in the
brain, which are a hallmark of
Alzheimer's disease.

Anticancer agent: Methylene
blue has also been studied for its
potential as an anticancer agent.
Some research has shown that

methylene blue may be effective in targeting and killing cancer cells, particularly in combination with other cancer treatments.

Antioxidant: Methylene blue has been shown to have antioxidant properties, which means it may help to protect against oxidative damage and inflammation in the body. Some research has suggested that methylene blue may be beneficial for the treatment of conditions such as sepsis and acute lung injury, which are characterized by inflammation and oxidative stress.

Wound healing: Methylene blue has been studied for its potential to promote wound healing. Some research has suggested that methylene blue may help to improve blood flow and oxygenation in wounded tissue, which can aid in the healing process.

Antiviral agent: Methylene blue has been shown to have antiviral properties, particularly against certain types of viruses such as HIV and herpes simplex virus. Some research has suggested that methylene blue may be effective in preventing the replication of these viruses and reducing their infectivity.

Memory enhancement:
Methylene blue has been studied for its potential to enhance memory and cognitive function, particularly in older adults. Some research has suggested that methylene blue may help to improve memory and cognitive function by increasing blood flow and oxygenation in the brain.

Antibiotic resistance: Methylene blue has been studied for its potential to combat antibiotic resistance, which is a growing problem in healthcare. Some research has suggested that methylene blue may be effective in enhancing the activity of certain antibiotics and preventing the development of resistance.

Energy production: Methylene blue has been studied for its potential to improve energy production in cells, particularly in patients with mitochondrial disorders. Some research has suggested that methylene blue may help to improve energy production by increasing the activity of certain enzymes involved in cellular respiration.

While the potential applications of methylene blue outlined above are promising, it is important to note that many of these uses are still in the experimental stages and have not been fully tested in humans. As with any new treatment or application, further research and testing will be necessary to fully understand its effectiveness, safety, and potential risks.

CHAPTER 4

Methylene Blue Dosage

The appropriate dosage of methylene blue depends on several factors including the intended use, the individual's age and weight, and any underlying health conditions. Here are some general guidelines for methylene blue dosage based on its different uses:

Diagnostic purposes: For diagnostic purposes, such as staining biological tissues for microscopy, methylene blue is typically used at a concentration of 1-2%. The exact amount used will depend on the specific staining protocol being used.

Treatment of methemoglobinemia: Methylene blue is used to treat methemoglobinemia, a condition in which the blood cannot effectively transport oxygen. The dosage of methylene blue for this purpose typically ranges from 1-2 mg/kg of body weight, administered intravenously over 5-10 minutes. This may be repeated as needed, based on the severity of the condition.

Treatment of cyanide poisoning: Methylene blue is sometimes

used as an antidote for cyanide poisoning, a potentially life-threatening condition. The dosage of methylene blue for this purpose varies depending on the severity of the poisoning and the individual's weight. A typical dose may be 1-2 mg/kg of body weight, administered intravenously over 5-10 minutes. This may be repeated as needed, based on the individual's response.

Treatment of malaria: Methylene blue is sometimes used as an alternative treatment for malaria, particularly in cases of drug-resistant strains. The dosage of methylene blue for this purpose typically ranges from 15-20 mg/kg of body weight, administered orally or intravenously over several days.

Other therapeutic uses: For other therapeutic uses, such as the treatment of septic shock, Alzheimer's disease, or cancer, the dosage of methylene blue will depend on the specific treatment protocol being used. Dosages may range from 1-10 mg/kg of body weight, administered orally or intravenously, and may be given once daily or multiple times per week.

It is important to note that methylene blue should always be administered under the supervision of a healthcare provider, as improper dosages or administration can lead to serious side effects. Additionally, the appropriate dosage of methylene blue may be affected by individual factors such as age, weight, and underlying health conditions, so it is important to follow the guidance of a healthcare provider when determining the appropriate dosage for a particular use.

The dosage of methylene blue varies depending on the intended use, individual factors such as age and weight, and any underlying health conditions. While guidelines exist for certain uses of methylene blue, it is important to always follow the guidance of a healthcare provider and to use caution when administering this compound.

CHAPTER 5

Properties that Methylene Blue

Methylene blue is a highly versatile and useful compound that possesses several unique chemical and physical properties. These properties make it useful for a variety of applications, including diagnostic purposes, therapeutic uses, and research applications. Here are some of the key properties of methylene blue:

Chemical structure: Methylene blue is a heterocyclic aromatic compound with a molecular formula of C16H18ClN3S. It contains a nitrogen atom within a fused ring structure that gives it its characteristic blue color. Methylene blue has a molecular weight of 319.85 g/mol and a melting point of 100-105°C.

Solubility: Methylene blue is highly soluble in water and forms a deep blue solution when dissolved. It is also soluble in ethanol, but is less soluble in other organic solvents.

Redox properties: Methylene blue is a redox-active compound, meaning that it can accept and donate electrons. This property makes it useful for a variety of diagnostic and therapeutic applications, including the treatment of methemoglobinemia and cyanide poisoning.

Photodynamic properties: Methylene blue is also known for its photodynamic properties, which allow it to absorb and emit light energy when exposed to certain wavelengths of light. This property makes it useful for a variety of research applications, such as photodynamic therapy and fluorescence microscopy.

Antimicrobial properties: Methylene blue has been shown to possess antimicrobial properties, particularly against certain bacteria and fungi. This property has led to its use as a topical antiseptic, as well as in the treatment of infections such as leishmaniasis.

Mitochondrial targeting: Recent research has shown that methylene blue can selectively target and accumulate in mitochondria, the cellular organelles responsible for energy production. This property has led to its investigation as a potential treatment for mitochondrial disorders, as well as its potential to enhance cellular energy production.

Absorption spectrum: Methylene blue has a characteristic absorption spectrum, which allows it to be easily detected and quantified using spectrophotometry. Its absorption spectrum is in the visible range, with a peak at around 660 nm.

Oxidation state: Methylene blue can exist in two different oxidation states: a reduced form, known as leucomethylene blue, and an oxidized form, known as methylene blue. These different oxidation states are important for its therapeutic and diagnostic uses, as the reduced form is used to treat methemoglobinemia, while the oxidized form is used for diagnostic staining.

pH sensitivity: Methylene blue is pH-sensitive, meaning that its color and solubility can be affected by changes in pH. It is most soluble and has its characteristic blue color at a pH of around 4-5.

Staining properties: Methylene blue is a highly effective stain and can be used to stain a variety of biological materials, including cells, tissues, and microorganisms. Its staining properties are based on its ability to interact with negatively charged components of cells and tissues, such as nucleic acids and proteins.

Optical properties: Methylene blue has interesting optical properties that make it useful for certain applications. For example, it is highly fluorescent, meaning that it can emit light when excited by a light source. This property has led to its use in fluorescence microscopy, where it can be used to label and visualize specific molecules or structures within cells.

Electron-transfer properties: Methylene blue is also known for its electron-transfer properties, which allow it to participate in certain biochemical reactions. For example, it can be used as a redox indicator to monitor changes in electron-transfer reactions, or as an electron acceptor in photosynthesis.

Oxidative stress response: Recent research has shown that methylene blue can also act as an antioxidant, protecting cells from oxidative stress. This property has led to its investigation as a potential treatment for neurodegenerative diseases such as Alzheimer's and Parkinson's, which are associated with oxidative stress and mitochondrial dysfunction

CHAPTER 6

Methylene Blue as a Neuroprotective Agent

Methylene blue has shown potential as a neuroprotective agent in a number of preclinical and clinical studies. Its neuroprotective effects are thought to be mediated by a number of mechanisms, including its ability to scavenge free radicals, inhibit mitochondrial dysfunction, and modulate neuronal signaling pathways.

One of the most well-studied potential uses of methylene blue as a neuroprotective agent is in the treatment of neurodegenerative diseases such as Alzheimer's and Parkinson's. These diseases are characterized by the progressive loss of neurons in certain regions of the brain, leading to cognitive and motor dysfunction.

Methylene blue has been shown to improve cognitive function and slow the progression of Alzheimer's disease in animal models. One study found that treatment with methylene blue reduced the accumulation of amyloid-beta plaques in the brains of mice with Alzheimer's disease, while also improving cognitive function and reducing inflammation.

In Parkinson's disease, methylene blue has been shown to protect against dopaminergic neuron loss and reduce the formation of toxic protein aggregates. One study found that methylene blue treatment improved motor function and reduced oxidative stress in a mouse model of Parkinson's disease.

methylene blue has also been investigated for its potential as a treatment for traumatic brain injury (TBI). TBI is a major cause of disability and death worldwide and is associated with a range of neurological deficits, including cognitive impairment, motor dysfunction, and psychiatric symptoms.

Studies have shown that methylene blue treatment can reduce brain damage and improve cognitive and motor function in animal models of TBI. For example, one study found that methylene blue treatment improved learning and memory function in rats following TBI, while also reducing brain inflammation and oxidative stress.

The exact mechanisms by which methylene blue exerts its neuroprotective effects are not fully understood. However, it is thought to act through a number of different pathways, including its ability to scavenge free radicals, inhibit mitochondrial dysfunction, and modulate neuronal signaling pathways.

CHAPTER 7

Methylene Blue for Stain Removal

Methylene blue is not only used in medicine, but also in other industries such as textile and laboratory science. In textile industry, it is often used as a dye and stain remover due to its ability to bind with organic molecules and remove them from fabrics.

The process of using methylene blue for stain removal involves soaking the stained fabric in a solution containing methylene blue. The solution can be made by dissolving methylene blue powder in water or other solvents such as ethanol. The fabric is then allowed to soak in the solution for a period of time, typically ranging from a few minutes to several hours, depending on the severity of the stain and the type of fabric.

Methylene blue works by binding to organic molecules in the stain, such as proteins, fats, and other complex molecules, and removing them from the fabric. This process is known as adsorption, and it occurs when the methylene blue molecules attach themselves to the organic molecules in the stain, forming a complex that can then be washed away from the fabric.

Methylene blue is particularly effective at removing stains from fabrics that are difficult to clean with traditional methods. For example, it can be used to remove blood stains from clothing, which can be notoriously difficult to remove with ordinary detergent and water. It can also be used to remove stains from delicate fabrics such as silk, which can be easily damaged by harsh chemicals.

One of the advantages of using methylene blue for stain removal is that it is relatively safe and non-toxic. Unlike some other stain removal agents, such as bleach or ammonia, methylene blue is not corrosive and does not produce harmful fumes. This makes it a popular choice for use in household cleaning products and other applications where safety is a concern.

However, it is important to note that methylene blue can stain fabrics if it is not used properly. This is because the dye can bind to the fabric itself, rather than the stain, resulting in a blue discoloration. Therefore, it is important to follow proper procedures when using methylene blue for stain removal, such as using the appropriate concentration of solution and avoiding prolonged exposure to the fabric. Additionally, it is important to wear protective gloves and clothing when handling methylene blue, as it can stain skin and clothing.

Methylene blue is a versatile dye and stain remover that is used in a variety of applications. In the textile industry, it is commonly used to dye cotton, silk, and other fabrics, as well as to remove stains from these materials. It is particularly effective at removing protein-based stains, such as blood, urine, and sweat, as well as stains from dyes and inks.

When used as a dye, methylene blue penetrates the fibers of the fabric and binds to the molecular structure of the fibers themselves. This produces a long-lasting and uniform color that is resistant to fading. The intensity of the color can be controlled by varying the concentration of the methylene blue solution and the length of time that the fabric is soaked in the dye bath.

When used as a stain remover, methylene blue works by binding to the organic molecules in the stain and removing them from the fabric. The dye molecules attach themselves to the stains through a process known as adsorption, in which they form weak chemical bonds with the molecules in the stain. The dye-stain complex is then washed away from the fabric during the rinse cycle.

Methylene blue is particularly effective at removing protein-based stains because it has a high affinity for these molecules. It is also effective at removing dye stains because it can break down the molecular structure of the dye and make it easier to remove from the fabric.

CHAPTER 8

Methylene Blue use as Anti-aging agent

There is not enough scientific evidence to support the claim that methylene blue can be used as an anti-aging agent. While some studies have suggested that methylene blue may have anti-aging properties, the evidence is limited and further research is needed to fully understand its potential benefits and risks.

Methylene blue is a synthetic compound that has been used for a variety of medical and nonmedical purposes for over a century. It has been studied for its potential to treat a range of conditions, including malaria, sepsis, and Alzheimer's disease. In recent years, there has been interest in its potential as an anti-aging agent due to its ability to affect cellular processes that are believed to contribute to aging.

One of the proposed mechanisms by which methylene blue may exert its anti-aging effects is through its ability to increase mitochondrial function. Mitochondria are the energy-producing organelles within cells, and their dysfunction is believed to contribute to aging and age-related diseases. Some studies have suggested that methylene blue can improve mitochondrial function by increasing the production of ATP, the primary energy currency of the cell.

To its effects on mitochondrial function, methylene blue has been shown to have antioxidant and anti-inflammatory properties, which may also contribute to its potential anti-aging effects. Oxidative stress and chronic inflammation are believed to be key drivers of aging and age-related diseases, and compounds that can reduce these processes may have anti-aging effects.

Despite these potential mechanisms, there is limited evidence to support the use of methylene blue as an anti-aging agent in humans. Most of the studies conducted on methylene blue and aging have been performed in animals or in vitro, and the results have been mixed.

For example, a study published in the journal Nature in 2016 found that methylene blue increased the lifespan of fruit flies by up to 40%. The researchers suggested that this was due to the compound's ability to increase mitochondrial function and reduce oxidative stress. However, it is important to note that the study was conducted in fruit flies, and it is unclear whether the same effects would be seen in humans.

Similarly, a study published in the journal Scientific Reports in 2017 found that methylene blue increased the lifespan of mice and improved their cognitive function. However, the study was small and used a high dose of methylene blue, which may not be safe for human use.

There have been a few studies conducted on the use of methylene blue in humans for age-related conditions, such as Alzheimer's disease. For example, a study published in the journal Frontiers in Aging

Neuroscience in 2014 found that methylene blue improved cognitive function in patients with Alzheimer's disease. However, the study was small and did not look specifically at the anti-aging effects of methylene blue.

while there is some evidence to suggest that methylene blue may have anti-aging properties, the evidence is limited and further research is needed to fully understand its potential benefits and risks. It is also important to note that methylene blue is a synthetic compound that can have side effects and may interact with other medications, so it should only be used under the supervision of a healthcare provider.

It is important to note that while methylene blue may have potential as an anti-aging agent, there are other factors that are known to play a much larger role in the aging process. These factors include genetics, lifestyle choices, and environmental exposures. While there is no way to completely stop the aging process, there are many steps that individuals can take to help maintain their health and vitality as they age.

Some of the most important steps that individuals can take to promote healthy aging include:

1. Eating a healthy diet: A diet that is rich in fruits, vegetables, whole grains, and lean protein can help support overall health and reduce the risk of chronic diseases that are associated with aging.

2. Staying physically active: Regular exercise can help maintain muscle mass, improve balance and flexibility, and reduce the risk of chronic diseases like heart disease and diabetes.

3. Getting enough sleep: Good quality sleep is essential for overall health and wellbeing, and can help

reduce the risk of age-related cognitive decline.

4. Managing stress: Chronic stress has been linked to a range of health problems, including heart disease, depression, and cognitive decline. Finding healthy ways to manage stress, such as through exercise, meditation, or spending time in nature, can help promote healthy aging.

5. Avoiding smoking and excessive alcohol consumption: Both smoking and excessive alcohol consumption have been linked to a range of

health problems, including cancer, heart disease, and cognitive decline.

While methylene blue may have potential as an anti-aging agent, it is important to approach any claims with caution and to rely on scientific evidence to guide decisions about its use. It is also important to take a holistic approach to healthy aging, focusing on overall health and wellbeing rather than a single compound or treatment. By taking steps to maintain a healthy lifestyle and seeking medical advice when necessary, individuals can help promote healthy aging and enjoy a long and fulfilling life.

CHAPTER 9

Methylene Blue as Anti Malaria Agent

Malaria is a serious and potentially life-threatening disease that is caused by the Plasmodium parasite. The disease is transmitted through the bites of infected mosquitoes and is particularly common in tropical and subtropical regions around the world. While there are a number of drugs available to treat and prevent malaria, there is still a great need for new and effective treatments that can help reduce the burden of this disease.

One potential new treatment for malaria is methylene blue. Methylene blue is a synthetic dye that has been used for a wide range of medical purposes, including as a treatment for methemoglobinemia, a rare blood disorder. In recent years, researchers have become interested in the potential of methylene blue as an anti-malarial agent.

There are several reasons why methylene blue may be effective against malaria. One is that it has been shown to have antiparasitic properties, meaning that it can help kill the Plasmodium parasite that causes malaria. In addition, methylene blue has been shown to have a number of other properties that could make it effective against malaria, including anti-inflammatory and antioxidant effects.

A number of studies have been conducted to investigate the potential of methylene blue as an anti-malarial agent. In one study, researchers tested methylene blue against the Plasmodium falciparum parasite, which is responsible for the majority of malaria cases in sub-Saharan Africa. The researchers found that methylene blue was able to inhibit the growth of the parasite in both laboratory and animal models.

Other studies have focused on the potential of methylene blue to be used as a prophylactic, or preventative, treatment for malaria. In one study, researchers tested methylene blue against Plasmodium berghei, a parasite that infects rodents and is commonly used as a model for human malaria. The researchers found that methylene blue was able to prevent the development of the parasite in mice that were given the drug prior to infection.

While the results of these studies are promising, more research is needed to fully understand the potential of methylene blue as an anti-malarial agent.

It is important to note that methylene blue is not currently approved for use as an anti-malarial drug, and any use of the drug for this purpose should be done under the guidance of a qualified healthcare professional.

Despite these challenges, the potential of methylene blue as an anti-malarial agent is exciting and could provide a new tool in the fight against this devastating disease. With continued research and development, methylene blue may one day become an important part of the global effort to control and eliminate malaria.

methylene blue may also have other benefits in the context of the disease. For example, some studies have suggested that methylene blue could help reduce the severity of the symptoms of malaria, such as fever and inflammation.

One study published in the Journal of Pharmacology and Experimental Therapeutics found that methylene blue was able to reduce fever and inflammation in mice infected with Plasmodium berghei. The researchers suggested that these effects could be due to the drug's anti-inflammatory properties, which may help reduce the immune system's response to the parasite.

Another study, published in the Journal of Infectious Diseases, found that methylene blue was able to reduce the production of cytokines, which are small proteins that are involved in the immune response. In malaria, cytokine production can become dysregulated, leading to inflammation and other complications. By reducing cytokine production, methylene blue may be able to help reduce the severity of these complications.

while more research is needed to fully understand the potential of methylene blue as an anti-malarial agent, the existing studies suggest that it could be a promising new tool in the fight against this disease. With its broad range of therapeutic properties and relatively low cost, methylene blue may be an attractive option for use in low-resource settings where malaria is most prevalent.

It is important to note, however, that methylene blue is not without its limitations and potential side effects. Like all drugs, methylene blue can cause adverse reactions in some patients, including headache, nausea, vomiting, and low blood pressure. In addition, the drug can interact with certain medications, such as antidepressants and antipsychotics, which can increase the risk of serotonin syndrome, a potentially life-threatening condition.

Despite these potential risks, the potential benefits of methylene blue in the context of malaria are significant, and continued research is needed to fully explore its potential as an anti-malarial agent. With further development and refinement, methylene blue may one day become an important tool in the global fight against malaria, helping to reduce the burden of this devastating disease and improve the lives of millions of people around the world.

Furthermore, some studies have also investigated the potential use of methylene blue in combination with other anti-malarial drugs. For example, one study published in the Journal of Antimicrobial Chemotherapy found that combining methylene blue with the anti-malarial drug artemisinin resulted in increased parasite clearance in mice infected with Plasmodium chabaudi. The researchers suggested that this combination therapy could potentially be used to reduce the development of drug resistance in the parasite, as well as improve the overall efficacy of anti-malarial treatment.

Another study, published in the American Journal of Tropical Medicine and Hygiene, found that adding methylene blue to the standard anti-malarial drug combination of artemether and lumefantrine resulted in improved clearance of Plasmodium falciparum in patients with uncomplicated malaria. The researchers suggested that the addition of methylene blue may have helped to overcome the resistance of the parasite to the standard anti-malarial drugs.

While these studies are promising, more research is needed to fully understand the potential of methylene blue as a combination therapy for malaria. it is important to note that the use of combination therapy for malaria is already standard practice in many areas, and the addition of methylene blue would need to be carefully evaluated to ensure that it is safe and effective.

CHAPTER 10

Benefits of Methylene Blue

Methylene blue is a versatile compound with a wide range of potential benefits across various fields. Here are some of the most notable benefits of methylene blue:

1. Antimicrobial properties: Methylene blue has been shown to have antimicrobial properties,

making it potentially useful in treating bacterial, viral, and fungal infections. It has been found to be effective against a variety of pathogens, including Staphylococcus aureus, Pseudomonas aeruginosa, Escherichia coli, Candida albicans, and herpes simplex virus.

2. Antioxidant properties: Methylene blue has antioxidant properties, which means it can help protect cells from damage caused by free radicals and oxidative stress. This property is believed to be one of the key mechanisms

by which methylene blue provides neuroprotective benefits.

3. Neuroprotective properties: Methylene blue has been shown to have neuroprotective properties, making it potentially useful in treating neurodegenerative diseases such as Alzheimer's and Parkinson's. It has been found to inhibit the aggregation of beta-amyloid protein, which is associated with the development of Alzheimer's disease, as well as to protect dopamine-producing neurons in the

brain, which are affected in Parkinson's disease.

4. Anti-aging properties: Methylene blue has been shown to have anti-aging properties, potentially due to its ability to improve mitochondrial function. Mitochondria are the powerhouses of the cells, and their dysfunction is believed to contribute to the aging process. Methylene blue has been found to improve mitochondrial respiration and increase the production of ATP, the primary source of energy for the cells.

5. Anti-inflammatory properties: Methylene blue has anti-inflammatory properties, which means it can help reduce inflammation throughout the body. This property is believed to be one of the key mechanisms by which methylene blue provides cardioprotective benefits.

6. Cardioprotective properties: Methylene blue has been shown to have cardioprotective properties, making it potentially useful in treating heart disease. It has been found to reduce oxidative stress and inflammation in the heart,

as well as to improve cardiac function and reduce the risk of arrhythmias.

7. Anti-malarial properties: Methylene blue has been shown to have anti-malarial properties, making it potentially useful in treating and preventing malaria. It has been found to inhibit the growth and replication of the Plasmodium parasite, which causes malaria.

8. Stain removal properties: Methylene blue is commonly used as a stain in biology and histology laboratories, and it also has

stain removal properties. It can be used to remove stains from fabrics, including those caused by blood and ink.

CHAPTER 11

Methylene Blue as an Antioxidant Properties

Methylene blue has been shown to have significant antioxidant properties, which can provide a variety of benefits to the body. Here are some of the ways in which methylene blue acts as an antioxidant:

1. Scavenging free radicals: Methylene blue has the ability to scavenge free

radicals, which are highly reactive molecules that can damage cells and tissues by oxidizing cellular components such as DNA, proteins, and lipids. By neutralizing free radicals, methylene blue can prevent oxidative stress and protect cells from damage.

2. Enhancing mitochondrial function: Methylene blue has been shown to improve mitochondrial function by increasing the production of ATP, the primary source of energy for cells. This can help reduce oxidative stress and prevent mitochondrial dysfunction, which is

believed to be a key factor in the development of many age-related diseases.

3. Protecting against lipid peroxidation: Methylene blue has been shown to protect against lipid peroxidation, which is the oxidation of lipids that can cause cellular damage and lead to the development of diseases such as Alzheimer's and Parkinson's. By preventing lipid peroxidation, methylene blue can help protect cells from damage and reduce the risk of disease.

4. Inhibiting protein aggregation: Methylene blue has been found to inhibit the aggregation of beta-amyloid protein, which is associated with the development of Alzheimer's disease. By preventing the aggregation of this protein, methylene blue can help protect neurons from damage and slow the progression of the disease.

5. Reducing inflammation: Methylene blue has been shown to have anti-inflammatory properties, which can help reduce oxidative stress and prevent

damage to cells and tissues. Inflammation is a key factor in the development of many chronic diseases, and by reducing inflammation, methylene blue can help protect against these diseases.

6. Promoting cellular regeneration: Methylene blue has been shown to promote the regeneration of cells by increasing the production of stem cells and promoting cell growth and division. This can help repair damaged cells and tissues and prevent the development of age-related diseases.

methylene blue's antioxidant properties make it a promising candidate for the prevention and treatment of a variety of diseases and conditions. By scavenging free radicals, enhancing mitochondrial function, protecting against lipid peroxidation, inhibiting protein aggregation, reducing inflammation, and promoting cellular regeneration, methylene blue can help protect against oxidative stress and promote overall health and wellbeing. However, more research is needed to fully understand the mechanisms by which methylene blue acts as an antioxidant and to determine the optimal dosages and administration routes for specific applications.

7. Improving cognitive function: Methylene blue has been shown to improve cognitive function, particularly in the areas of memory and attention. This is likely due in part to its ability to protect against oxidative stress and inflammation, which can damage neurons and impair cognitive function.

8. Reducing the risk of cardiovascular disease: Methylene blue has been

shown to improve cardiovascular function by increasing blood flow, reducing oxidative stress, and protecting against inflammation. This can help reduce the risk of cardiovascular disease and improve overall cardiovascular health.

9. Treating cyanide poisoning: Methylene blue is also used as an antidote for cyanide poisoning, which can occur from exposure to smoke inhalation, industrial chemicals, or certain medications. Methylene blue works by converting cyanide to a less toxic form

that can be excreted from the body.

10.   Treating methemoglobinemia: Methylene blue is also used to treat methemoglobinemia, a condition in which the blood is unable to carry enough oxygen due to the presence of methemoglobin, a form of hemoglobin that cannot bind to oxygen. Methylene blue works by converting methemoglobin back to normal hemoglobin, allowing it to bind to oxygen and deliver it to the body's tissues.

11.   Treating urinary tract infections: Methylene blue has been shown to have antibacterial properties and may be effective in treating urinary tract infections caused by certain bacteria.

12.   Treating sepsis: Methylene blue has been shown to be effective in treating sepsis, a life-threatening condition that occurs when the body's response to an infection causes inflammation and damage to tissues and organs. Methylene blue works by reducing inflammation and improving cardiovascular

function, which can help prevent organ failure and improve outcomes for patients with sepsis.

Overall, methylene blue's antioxidant properties make it a promising candidate for a wide range of applications, from treating age-related diseases and cognitive decline to improving cardiovascular function and treating acute medical emergencies. However, more research is needed to fully understand its mechanisms of action and determine the optimal dosages and administration routes for specific applications.

13.   Treating Parkinson's disease: Methylene blue has also shown potential as a treatment for Parkinson's disease, a neurodegenerative disorder characterized by the loss of dopamine-producing neurons in the brain. Methylene blue works by inhibiting the aggregation of alpha-synuclein, a protein that is involved in the development of Parkinson's disease.

14.   Treating Alzheimer's disease: Methylene blue has also been studied for its potential in treating Alzheimer's disease, a

neurodegenerative disorder characterized by the accumulation of beta-amyloid plaques and tau protein tangles in the brain. Methylene blue has been shown to reduce the accumulation of beta-amyloid plaques and improve cognitive function in animal models of Alzheimer's disease.

15.   Enhancing exercise performance: Methylene blue has been shown to enhance exercise performance by improving the body's ability to use oxygen and reduce muscle fatigue. This makes it a

promising supplement for athletes and individuals looking to improve their physical performance.

16.   Improving wound healing: Methylene blue has been shown to improve wound healing by increasing blood flow and promoting the growth of new blood vessels, which can help deliver oxygen and nutrients to the site of the wound and promote tissue regeneration.

17.   Preventing kidney damage: Methylene blue has been shown to prevent kidney damage by reducing

oxidative stress and inflammation, which can be caused by certain medications or medical procedures.

18.   Preventing liver damage: Methylene blue has also been shown to prevent liver damage by reducing oxidative stress and inflammation, which can be caused by toxins or alcohol consumption.

19.   Treating mitochondrial disorders: Methylene blue has been studied for its potential in treating mitochondrial disorders, a group of

genetic disorders that affect the function of the mitochondria, the cells' energy producers. Methylene blue works by enhancing mitochondrial function and reducing oxidative stress, which can help improve symptoms in individuals with mitochondrial disorders.

20.   Promoting hair growth: Methylene blue has been shown to promote hair growth by increasing blood flow to hair follicles and stimulating the growth of new hair cells.

These are just a few of the potential benefits of methylene blue. However, it is important to note that many of these applications are still in the early stages of research and more studies are needed to determine their effectiveness and safety in humans. As with any supplement or medication, it is important to consult with a healthcare professional before using methylene blue for any purpose.

CHAPTER 12

Adverse Effect of Methylene Blue

While methylene blue has a wide range of potential benefits, it can also have adverse effects, especially at high doses or when used improperly. Some of the most common adverse effects of methylene blue include:

1. Headache: One of the most common side effects of methylene blue is headache, which can range from mild to severe.

2. Nausea and vomiting: Methylene blue can also cause nausea and vomiting, which may be more common when the drug is administered intravenously.

3. Abdominal pain: Some people may experience abdominal pain or discomfort after taking methylene blue.

4. Diarrhea: Methylene blue can cause diarrhea in some

people, especially when taken in high doses.

5. Dizziness: Methylene blue can cause dizziness or lightheadedness, which can increase the risk of falls and other accidents.

6. Low blood pressure: In some cases, methylene blue can cause a sudden drop in blood pressure, which can lead to fainting or shock.

7. Methemoglobinemia: Methemoglobinemia is a potentially life-threatening condition that can occur when methylene blue is used improperly or in high doses. This condition

occurs when methylene blue reacts with hemoglobin in the blood, reducing its ability to transport oxygen. Symptoms of methemoglobinemia may include shortness of breath, rapid heart rate, and blue or gray skin color.

8. Allergic reactions: Some people may have an allergic reaction to methylene blue, which can cause symptoms such as itching, rash, and difficulty breathing.

9. Interactions with other drugs: Methylene blue can interact with other drugs,

including certain antidepressants and antipsychotics, increasing the risk of adverse effects.

10.   Kidney damage: In rare cases, methylene blue can cause kidney damage, especially when used in high doses or for extended periods of time.

11.   Photosensitivity: Methylene blue can cause photosensitivity, which makes the skin more sensitive to sunlight. This can lead to sunburn, skin rash, and other skin irritations.

12.   Electrolyte imbalances: Methylene blue can cause electrolyte imbalances, particularly when used in high doses. This can result in symptoms such as muscle weakness, cramps, and irregular heartbeats.

13.   Methemoglobinemia in infants: Methylene blue should not be used in infants under three months of age, as they are at a higher risk of developing methemoglobinemia. Symptoms of methemoglobinemia in infants may include bluish-

gray skin, seizures, and difficulty breathing.

14.   Psychological effects: In rare cases, methylene blue can cause psychological effects, including confusion, agitation, and hallucinations.

15.   Hemolysis: Hemolysis is the destruction of red blood cells, which can occur when methylene blue is used in high doses or for extended periods of time. Symptoms of hemolysis may include jaundice,

fatigue, and shortness of breath.

16.   Interactions with other medications: Methylene blue can interact with other medications, particularly those used to treat depression and anxiety. Combining methylene blue with certain antidepressants can lead to a dangerous condition called serotonin syndrome, which can cause symptoms such as high fever, seizures, and rapid heart rate.

17.   Allergic reactions: Some people may be allergic to methylene blue.

Symptoms of an allergic reaction may include rash, hives, itching, swelling, and difficulty breathing.

18.   Gastrointestinal disturbances: Methylene blue can cause gastrointestinal disturbances, such as nausea, vomiting, and diarrhea.

19.   Urine discoloration: Methylene blue can turn urine blue or green, which can be alarming but is generally harmless.

20.   Other potential side effects: Methylene blue may cause other potential

side effects, such as headache, dizziness, and fatigue.

It is important to note that many of these adverse effects are rare and may only occur at high doses or when methylene blue is used improperly. However, it is still important to use methylene blue under the guidance of a healthcare professional and to monitor for any potential side effects. If you experience any adverse effects while taking methylene blue, it is important to seek medical attention right away.